EPILEPSY AWARENESS

"The struggles of living with Epilepsy"

Ch.1) The Beginning

Epilepsy comes and goes at different stages of all our lives. Some of us are born with it; others don't end up getting diagnosed with it until later in life. Me personally, I've had epilepsy since I was five months old.

I know some people say it's always more tough in the beginning, that it'll get easier as time goes on. But in this case it depends on the situation and when exactly you got diagnosed with epilepsy.

If you're anything like me and you've had epilepsy since you were a young kid or since you were born, etc. then you might agree that it's easier in the beginning. Why? Because, yes were diagnosed with epilepsy and are having seizures back to back. BUT as babies or young kids were not the ones who have to deal with the responsibility that comes with it.

Call me crazy…but you'll understand when I'm finished. Obviously because were young kids with epilepsy and we can't help it. And were under eighteen so were not responsible for the things we are now to take care of ourselves and our condition.

But who is? You've got it. Our parents or for some might be a different parental figure...But you get the idea. Anyways they're the ones who were there to make sure we had our medicine as often as needed, that we ate 3x a day, got proper rest, took us to see our neurologist, etc. If anyone would say the beginning was rough it'd be them.

Now if you were diagnosed later in life then yes the beginning is gonna be rough. After I turned eighteen was the day I realized all the stress my parents went through having to raise a child that has epilepsy.

Being an adult and living with epilepsy, especially if you're an adult that's just been diagnosed with epilepsy. You're basically living around it. As a child you don't realize the things you do as an adult. Also, as a child the same things don't get you as they would when you're an adult.

Living with epilepsy can be either a rough or easy beginning. It all depends on what stage of your life you get diagnosed with it. But I can promise the fight is worth the battle cause the outcome will always be greater.

Ch.2) The Struggle

Just like cancer, or cystic fibrosis, even people with epilepsy have our issues and our everyday struggles.

Cancer patients lose their hair; Cystic fibrosis patients have lung problems and have to spend weeks in the hospital getting lung treatments. People like myself that have epilepsy, have a brain disorder that cause us to have seizures.

But there is so much more than that, that comes with Epilepsy than just seizures.

Epilepsy can interfere with our heart and breathing. It can cause shortness of breath, coughing, or sometimes choking. Over long periods of times Epilepsy can increase risk of heart disease or stroke.

Some of the drugs used to treat Epilepsy, can cause digestive problems such as heart burn, nausea, and even vomiting. Another problem can also be Constipation and Diarrhea. Epilepsy itself can cause abdominal pain.

Women that have epilepsy, that get pregnant have a 25-40 percent increased risk of having a seizure. There is also an increased risk of hypertension, delivering an underweight baby and still birth.

And those are just a few of the major issues that we may or may not have to worry about. Some of the issues or struggles we live with everyday are:

Feeling Dizzy or lightheaded- if you're anything like me that'll usually happen after getting to hot or being in the heat to long, getting up to fast, etc.

Feeling tired or sleepy- that will usually be a side effect of the medicine you're prescribed.

Double Vision or Blurry Vision- "Now I know why my eyes are so bad!"

Poor Coordination or balance- If you've ever been to your neurologist office and they make you walk in a straight line or heal to toe, this is why.

Unsteady Walking- "Are we drunk?"

Headache- This will also usually be another side effect of your prescribed medicine.

So as we can see there is so much more to living with epilepsy than just "seizures". So many people hear the word epilepsy and automatically assume it's just about seizures, But in reality there is so much more to it than that.

It's the random shaking we get when holding a glass, or watching t.v. It's the sleepless nights cause were too afraid to go to sleep cause we think

we're gonna have a seizure in our
sleep.

It's the nights we do wake up in the
middle of the night with our heart
racing and head pounding cause we
just got ourselves out of a seizure in
our sleep.

It's about the days where you're stuck
staying inside cause it's too hot out
and you don't want to have a seizure
from the heat.

It's about the times you wake up in the
ambulance cause you just had a
seizure and they won't pull over to let
you go to the bathroom. Epilepsy is

real. **You can't see it physically but the pain is still there. You can't see it. But we can feel it.**

Ch.3) Meeting New People

The look of fear you get when meeting new people is probably one of the hardest things to deal with when you live with epilepsy. Wither it's a job, boyfriend, girlfriend, or a random person you meet at the store.

They all assume the same thing…that if we have a seizure in front of them that it's the end of the world. They're not gonna know what to do, so they assume the next best thing is to run away.

Let me tell you this if you or someone you know has epilepsy. And you think they're gonna have a seizure in front of you…DON'T run. If you don't think you'd know what to do…then go get HELP right AWAY.

Especially if you don't feel comfortable helping someone that's having a seizure…then get help right AWAY. Don't run. And DON'T wait until after everything is said and done. Cause by then it could be too late.

BUT I can let you know firsthand that there's nothing to be afraid of as long as you stay calm. Cool. And collected.

The biggest mistake people make when hearing that someone has epilepsy, is trying to picture the image in their head, or imitate it based off of the image they put in their head.

When people hear the word epilepsy they automatically think about twitching, and "stupid". Because, we have Epilepsy and have seizures they assume were stupid. But anyone with Epilepsy, including myself can tell you that's not true. It's just a very big false assumption.

I've has people ask me if I act the way I do because of me having Epilepsy....do you think they're thinking that now? Bet not.

Anyways, having a seizure is more than just "twitching"; it also depends on the type of Epilepsy you've been diagnosed with. Depending on how serious your epilepsy is, will determine what kind've seizures you'll usually have. But we'll get deeper into that later on.

Usually, a seizure will consist of, shaking, twitching, foam coming out of our mouths, losing control of bladder, etc.

The best thing to do when any of these things happen is STAY CALM! If you notice any strange behavior then stay ALERT! PAY ATTENTION to the warning signs'1 Headaches, complaints about being too hot, Dizziness, Lightheaded, Vomiting, etc.

If any of the above symptoms are going on or more then stay by that person and be prepared to catch them. If they break out into a seizure then put them onto their side an start counting how long the seizure lasts. If it last longer than about a minute, Immediately call 911.

It's hard to trust a new person coming into our lives and having to explain to them what epilepsy is. And then trusting that they'll stick around afterwards. So, believe me when I say the most important thing you can do when someone who has epilepsy has a seizure in front of you, is to just comfort them and love them through it.

I can promise you that the same set of questions run through every epileptics mind when meeting someone new or a new employer,

"What are they gonna do if I have a seizure?", "What if I have a seizure at work?" ,"Will I get fired?", "Are they gonna have someone who knows what they're doing if I have a seizure?"

If you're meeting with an employer you need to get all of these questions answered before you take the job. Make sure there will be someone there to make sure you'll be taken care of if you have a seizure. Don't wait until the day you feel like you're gonna have one and end up falling on your head!

If you're meeting with a potential significant other or even a new friend you need to make sure they understand you have epilepsy. Make sure if they're gonna be apart of your life that they understand they can't just come in and walk back out as they please. Cause were epileptic and are fighting a battle just like cancer or diabetes. We need their love and comfort just as much.

Ch.4) Identifying The Cause

The most important thing in an epileptic's life is finding the reason they have epilepsy to begin with.

Why? Because we all wonder if we find the cause if we can fix that cause so we don't have to live with epilepsy anymore.

This is why we have to get EEGs and MRIs done, so our neurologist can see any abnormal brain activity going on that'll hopefully tell him/her why we have epilepsy. But we'll get more into that later.

If you're anything like me, then you're still searching for answers. Cause no matter how many EEGs or MRIs we've had they come back normal so we still don't know what's causing our epilepsy.

Is it coming from the left side of our brain or the right side? Or somewhere in the center?

I can guarantee you the same set of questions run through every person living with epilepsy mind.

If having just one beer puts me at higher risk for a seizure, then what causes that? Why do they know I shouldn't drink but can't tell me why I have epilepsy?

If stress is a trigger for our seizures then what causes that? Why do they know stress puts me at a higher risk for a seizure but can't tell me why I have epilepsy?

Strobe Lights…were not supposed to be around strobe lights. Cause it's flashing sensors can trigger us to have a seizure, Right? Why do they know that, but not the cause of why we have epilepsy?

The Heat…hot showers, hot temperatures, hot working environments, etc. They're all a trigger for us to have a seizure right? Why do they know that but they can't tell us what our cause is for having epilepsy.

These and so many more, make us question our neurologist, Dr, etc. I'm sure most that live with epilepsy can agree with me. And if not I bet you are now.

Think about it. We deserve answers. If we knew what were the cause behind our epilepsy then maybe we could fix that cause. And if we fix that cause then maybe we could stop living behind closed closed doors or with an invisible shield in front of us.

Because, another important thing to those living with epilepsy is keeping ourselves protected. And there are two ways to do that.

Those that don't have their epilepsy under control stay behind closed doors. Without the meds to keep them under control, they don't wanna risk anything they don't have to. Why? As if having epilepsy isn't scary enough so will that medical bill be if something were to happen. So they shelter theirsleves the best they can. And if something happens while their home, they don't call 911 unless they feel they have no other choice.

Now, for those who do have their epilepsy under control, they tend to hold up a invisible shield. Thinking it'll protect them from the outside looking in.

Even though myself, along with many others have their epilepsy under control a little better than those who don't, it doesn't mean that were not as afraid of something happening as they are.

So, in conclusion my point being that if we all knew what the cause of our epilepsy were, where it was coming from, then maybe we wouldn't need to his behind closed doors, or put up invisible shields.

Cause if we found out the cause of our epilepsy, then we'd be able to protect ourselves the right way, Instead of protecting ourselves from the outside world.

We deserve answers, not to keep waiting another twenty one years, and getting EEGs and MRIs done every six months to a year and getting no results.

If they can tell us all our triggers to our seizures and tell us what to expect taking a certain medicine. Then why are they making us wait to find the cause for our epilepsy?

We deserve to know, not to ask ourselves "What if we never find out."

Ch.5) Different Types of Epilepsy/Seizures

One thing people make the mistake of is thinking Epilepsy is just "Epilepsy".

First of all let me break it down to you what epilepsy actually is, and then I'll talk about the different types of epilepsy and seizures that come with it.

Epilepsy is the occurrence of sporadic electrical storms in the brain commonly called seizures. These storms cause behavioral manifestations (such as staring) or involuntary movements (such as grand mal seizures).

There are several different types of epilepsy, each have different causes, symptoms, and treatments.

When making a diagnosis of epilepsy, your neurologist may use one of the following terms: Idiopathic, Cryptogenic, Symptomatic, Generalized, Focal, or Partial. Idiopathic means there is no apparent cause. Cryptogenic means there is a likely cause but has not been identified. Generalized means the seizures are involving the whole brain at once. Focal or Partial means that the seizure is starting from one area of the brain.

The major types of epilepsy are:

-Idiopathic (genetic causes)

-Symptomatic (cause unknown) or Cryptogenic (cause unknown)

-Generalized Epilepsy

-Childhood Absence Epilepsy

-Juvenile myoclonic epilepsy

-Epilepsy with grand-mal seizures on awakening others

-West syndrome

-Lennox-Gastaut syndrome

-Temporal lobe syndrome

-Frontal lobe syndrome

Now that you know what epilepsy is and all the major kinds of epilepsy…Now I will break down each one for you.

Idiopathic Generalized Epilepsy- In this type of epilepsy, there is often, but not always a family history of epilepsy, it tends to appear during childhood or adolescence, although it may not be diagnosed until adulthood. In this type of epilepsy no nervous system (brain or spinal cord) abnormalities other than seizures can be identified on either EEG or MRI. Special studies may show a scar or subtle change in the brain that may have been present since birth.

The results of the electroencephalogram (EEG a test which measures electrical impulses in the brain) may show epileptic discharge affecting a single area or multiple areas in the brain (so called generalized discharges).

The types of seizures affecting patients with idiopathic generalized epilepsy may include:

- Myoclonic seizures (sudden and very short duration jerking of the extremities)
- Absence seizures AKA staring spells
- Generalized tonic-clonic seizures (grand mal seizures)

Idiopathic generalized epilepsy is usually treated with medications. Some people outgrow this condition and stop having seizures, as in the case with childhood absence epilepsy and a large number of patients with juvenile myoclonic epilepsy.

Idiopathic Partial Epilepsy- This type of epilepsy begins between ages 5-8 of our childhood, and may even be part of a family history. It's also known as benign focal epilepsy of childhood (BFEC); This is considered one of the mildest types of epilepsy. It is almost always outgrown by puberty and is never diagnosed in adults.

For this type of epilepsy seizures tend to occur during sleep and are often simple partial motor seizures that involve the face and secondarily generalized (grand-mal) seizures. Usually this type of epilepsy will be diagnosed with an EEG.

Symptomatic Generalized Epilepsy- This type of epilepsy is caused by widespread brain damage. Injury during birth is the most common cause of symptomatic generalized epilepsy. In addition to seizures these patients often have other neurological problems, such as mental retardation or cerebral palsy. Specific, inherited brain diseases, such as ADL or brain infections (such as meningitis and encephalitis) can also cause symptomatic generalized epilepsy.

When the cause of this type of epilepsy can't be identified, the disorder maybe referred to as cryptogenic epilepsy. These epilepsies include different subtypes the most commonly known type is the Lennox Gastaut syndrome.

Multiple types of seizures come along with this type of epilepsy such as: Generalized tonic-clonic, tonic, myoclonic, atonic and absence seizures. These are the most common in these patients and can be difficult to control.

Symptomatic Partial Epilepsy- Also known as Focal Epilepsy, it is the most common type of epilepsy that begins in adulthood. Although, it does frequently occur in children. This type of epilepsy is caused by a localized abnormality of the brain, which can result from strokes, tumors, trauma, congenital (present at birth) brain abnormality, scarring or "sclerosis" of brain tissue, cysts, or infections.

Sometimes these brain abnormalities can be seen on an MRI scan, but often they cannot be identified, despite repeated attempts, because they are "microscopic".

This type of epilepsy can be successfully treated with surgery that is aimed to remove he abnormal area without compromising the function of the rest of the brain. Epilepsy surgery is very successful in a large number of epilepsy patients who failed multiple anticonvulsant medications and who have identifiable lesions. These patients undergo a persurgical comprehensive epilepsy evaluation in dedicated and specialized epilepsy centers.

Now you know all the different types of epilepsy. You know the major kinds of epilepsy. And what they mean and the seizures that come along with it.

Now you know to never make the mistake again of thinking Epilepsy is just "Epilepsy". Cause it's so much more.

Ch.6) EEGs

As I've explained in previous chapters. One thing in a person that lives with epilepsy life is getting an EEG done to search for answers as to why we have epilepsy in the first place.

But sometimes it's not always about finding out just why we have epilepsy, sometimes it's just to make sure everything is ok, or to check our medicine levels, or sometimes our neurologist will order one after we've had a seizure to find out what happened. Especially if it were the first seizure we've had after a long period of time.

So, in this chapter we will discuss the different types of EEGs, what they are, and the purpose behind them.

An EEG is a test that they place electrodes (flat metal discs) on your head. That will pick up electrical signals from your brain and record them on the EEG machine.

The electrodes pick up the electrical signals. They do not affect your brain or cause any pain.

The EEG records the electrical signals from your brain on a computer. They look like wavy lines and represent your brainwave patterns. The EEG test can only show your brainwave patterns at the time the test is carried out, your brainwave patterns maybe different at different times.

Now that you know what an EEG actually is I will explain the different kinds of them that there are. So next time you, or someone you live with that has epilepsy says they have to get an EEG done, you can know what kind've EEG it is.

Standard EEG test- Usually, a standard EEG is done at a hospital with an appointment. It lasts between one and one and half hours. And you're safe to go home afterwards…It's not the dentist…you're not gonna be numb or swollen afterwards…I promise.

You'll either be sitting or lying down during the test. Whoever gives you your test will use a sticky gel to attach the electrodes to your head. You'll be asked to breathe deeply an look into a flashing light for a few minutes.

These activites can change the electrical activity in your brain, which will show on the computer. It'll also help the neurologist to make a diagnosis.

You'll be asked to keep as still as possible while all this is going on. Any sudden movement can change the electrical activity in your brain, which can affect results.

Sleep EEG test- Your neurologist may ask you to have an EEG test while you are asleep. This could be because your seizures happen when you are asleep or tired. Or, you may have had a standard EEG test when you were awake, but it didn't show any unusual electrical activity. When you're asleep, your brainwave patterns change and may show more unusually electrical activity.

A sleep EEG is usually done in a hospital using a standard EEG machine. Before, the test, you must be given some medicine to make you go to sleep. The test lasts for one to two hrs and you usually go home once you have woken up.

Sleep Deprived EEG test- This test is done when you have had less sleep than usual. When you are tired, there is more chance that there will be unusual electrical activity in your brain. Your neurologist may have you have this test done. If you have had a standard EEG test, but it didn't show any unusual electrical activity.

Before a sleep deprived EEG test, your doctor may ask you not to go to sleep at all the night before, or to wake up earlier than normal.

The beginning of an sleep deprived EEG is the same as a standard test. You may fall asleep or doze off while the EEG is still recording the activity in your brain. The test will last for a few hours and you may go home once you wake up.

Ambulatory EEG- Ambulatory means designed for walking. So you can have a Ambulatory EEG test while you are moving around. An Ambulatory EEG test is designed to record the activity in your brain over a few hours, days, or even weeks.

This means there is more chance that it will pick up epileptic activity in your brain, than during a standard EEG test.

For this test you don't need to go to the hospital for. You wear the machine on a belt, so you can go about your daily business. The only difference between these electrodes and the ones for a standard..Is, these electrodes for this test are plugged into a small machine that record the results.

Your neurologist will ask you to keep a diary of your activites, such as sleeping and eating, while you are wearing the ambulatory EEG. They will also ask you, or somebody who is with you, to keep a detailed record of any seizures you have. They will then be able to match up what has been happening with the results of your brainwave activity on the EEG test results.

Video-telemetry Tests- During a video telemetry test; you need to stay in the hospital. A video telemetry test involves wearing an ambulatory EEG. At the same time, all your movements are recorded by a video camera. The test is usually carried out over a few days. Sometimes your epilepsy medicine maybe reduced or withdrawn. This is to increase the chances that you will have a seizure that can be recorded.

After the test, doctors, can watch the video to see any seizures you had. They also can look at the EEG results for the time you were having the seizure. This will tell them about any changes to your brainwave patterns at the time of the seizure.

You usually only have a video telemetry test if you've already been diagnosed with epilepsy. Here are some examples of why your neurologist might ask for one:

- It isn't clear what type of seizures you have.
- Your epilepsy medicine isn't working well
- There is a possibility your seizures aren't caused by epilepsy but something else.

- You're considering epilepsy surgery.

Now you know what all the different types of EEGs are and what to expect and how to prepare for them. In the next chapter we will get even deeper talking about MRIs.

Ch.7)MRIs

In this chapter we will look close at MRIs, what they are, and how they can help those living with epilepsy get the answers they're looking for.

MRI stands for magnetic resource imaging; it will not say for certain whether a person has epilepsy or not. But alongside other information, these might help the neurologist to decide if epilepsy is a likely cause of the seizures.

MRI is a technique which is used to create an image or scan of the brain. MRI scans can be used to look at the structure of the person's brain (how their brain is made up). In people with epilepsy it can be used to see if there is an obvious reason (structural cause) for their seizures. This might be a scar or lesion on their brain that can be seen on the image. However, many people have brain lesions without epilepsy, and many people with epilepsy do not have any scar or lesions on the brain.

So, How does MRI work?
Basically…the MRI scanner uses magnetic fields and radio waves to create an image of the brain.
But…it's not that simple…of course!

There's the science behind it..The Atoms and Protons. Boring? Maybe. But to understand how MRI works, we need to know a little bit about the tiny particles that make up the cells in our bodies. Atoms are the tiny particles which makeup all types of matter and everyday objects. Atoms themselves are made up of three even tinier particles called protons, neutrons, and electrons, makeup the atoms nucleus (centre), which is surrounded by the electrons.

The human body is mainly made up of water, and water contains hydrogen atoms. Hydrogen atoms have a special property known as spin, which is like a tiny magnetic field. MRI works by using this property of hydrogen atoms. This means that the nucleus of each hydrogen atom responds to radio waves that are produced by the MRI scanner, and this causes the nuclei to produce an MRI signal.

So, why is knowing all this important? At the centre of the MRI scanner is a strong magnet, made up of coils of wire. And electrical current is passed through the coils to create a magnetic field. The coils are often supercooled (cooled to a very low temperature) This means that the magnetic field created by the scanner is always switched on.

At the start of the scan the person having the scan will be moved inside the scanner. The scanner will usually be shaped like a cylinder or tube, the person lies inside the tube, inside the coils of the magnet. At this point the nuclei of the hydrogen atoms in the body are not organized in any particular direction; they are randomly arranged.

Once inside the scanner, the magnetic field causes the nuclei in the body to line up in the same direction as the magnetic field (this is called the equilibrium position)

Next, radio waves (pulses of electromagnetic energy) are created by the MRI scanner. The energy is then absorbed by the nuclei in the body. Which causes them to move away from the direction they were lined up in (becoming disturbed from the equilibrium position)

The radio signals are then switched off. And the nuclei return to line up with the magnetic field again (returning to the equilibrium position) To do this, the nuclei release energy as radio waves. Different types of tissue in the body (such as muscles or the brain) are made of different substances and different densities. Because of this, the nuclei of different tissues return to equilibrium at different times. The radio waves produced by the nuclei are picked up and measured by the MRI scanner, and are used to create the picture of the body or brain.

How are these signals used to take a picture? Well…The MRI scanner uses a computer to make complicated calculations to generate a picture from the strength and location of the radio wave signals. The strength of the signal is shown as different shades of grey.

There are many different types of MRI scans; A person can get…using different type of radio frequency pulses, and these give different types of images.

Everything we've been talking about; has been about a functional MRI. Which is what a person with epilepsy will usually have to get most of the time your neurologist orders an MRI.

The other types of MRIs are: Spectroscopy,   DTI, tractrography, CT scan.

Having an MRI could help someone living with epilepsy get their answers better than an EEG could, is because as you can see after we've talked about both. An MRI goes deeper than a EEG does.

So, next time you have to have an MRI done, yes there is hope for answers. Yes, there is hope to find your reason for having epilepsy. Don't lose hope.

Ch.8) The Cans and Cannots

So many people make the mistake of treating Epilepsy as if it were a joke or as if it's not real…including us that do live with it. Those that don't live with it do this because they don't physically see the damage of epilepsy like you do cancer, or if someone got into a fight. So they think were faking and they make jokes. Now, those that do live with it, do this because we don't wanna accept it. We don't wanna hear we can't do something just because we have epilepsy. But it's not always about what you can't do it's about what you still can do.

So in this chapter, we will talk about both. So those who do and don't live with Epilepsy can give it the right attention. If you live with Epilepsy then this chapter will help you to know what you can do to help take better care of it. If you don't live it but know someone who does then this chapter will help you to better help that person.

First thing first…As epileptics we CAN live a normal life. People make the mistake of thinking that because we have epilepsy that we have to be sheltered from the outside world…NO that's the worst thing you can do! Because if you shelter yourself or someone with epilepsy then how will they ever know how to take care of theirsleves and know what to look out for?

We can go outside and do everyday things just like someone who doesn't have epilepsy can. BUT we can't get behind the wheel unless we have been seizure free for 6 months to a year. That's why you see so many people celebrating it when they do go that long without one. Especially an adult cause it means they can finally have their freedom...or have it back.

We can't drink...or we aren't supposed to anyways, I'm sure I'm not the only one who has taken the risk. But as my neurologist would say "Even just one beer can put you at higher risk for a seizure". So if you have epilepsy and your seizures aren't under control very well then I wouldn't put myself under that kind've risk.

We CAN work...As long as your seizures are under control then you're okay to work. But as we've talked about in previous chapters..if you're gonna work then be sure to tell your employer that you have epilepsy and get any questions you may have answered right then and there at the interview.

We can't eat whatever we want..No were not diabetic BUT your diet is said to be a cause to trigger a seizure. So if you're careful about what you eat and stay away from fatty foods and caffeine then it could just put you at lower risk for a seizure.

We can't play sports...or at least very few. Jogging, football, etc. have been proven to be very safe. But other sports such as swimming, skydiving, or sailing require supervision or shouldn't be done at all. When playing sports and living with epilepsy it is important to take the important steps to avoid sports related problems...such as dehydration, overexertion, and hypoglycemia.

We CAN get an education, just because we live with epilepsy doesn't mean it makes us any less capable of making something of ourselves. Statistics show that only 56% of people with epilepsy finish high school and only 15% finish college. And 25% of working age people with epilepsy are unemployed.

Don't you wanna make those percentages go up? Why are we afraid to show the world what were made of? We CAN be successful. If we stop being fearful of having a seizure and having a greater fear of being unsuccessful then we could be unstoppable.

Ch.9) The Blessing

But the thing to remember is that through this non-stop everyday battle we fight is that we are blessed. Why? Because, God has stuck by all of our sides and gotten us through our roughest days.

We wouldn't be where we are today without god on our side to wake us up every morning, and give us the strength to keep going. And the courage to do whatever it is we need or want to do that day.

Some people living with epilepsy experience a roller coaster of mixed emotions. Depression, Anxiety, etc. So for some it's just a blessing to have the motivation to get up and get out of bed and brush our teeth.

For some people living with epilepsy the blessing is being able to start a family and have healthy children cause they were afraid they weren't going to beable to.

For others the blessing could be finishing school cause they were afraid to originally cause they thought they were gonna be bullied for having epilepsy.

No matter what your blessing is, the biggest blessing of all that we all have in common is being alive and surviving this battle. We have epilepsy, epilepsy does not have us.